IN THE HEARTBEAT OF NOW

In the Heartbeat of Now

A Principal-Pastor's Guide to Overcoming Anxiety and Embracing the Present

ANTON ANTHONY ED.S, THD.

Anton Anthony Ed.S, ThD.

CONTENTS

INTRODUCTION: TWO WORLDS, ONE MISSION

Have you ever felt ensnared by relentless worries and uncertainties that threaten to consume your peace? As a child, the pressures may have been about fitting in, receiving that much-anticipated call from a sweetheart, or grappling with the elusive concept of popularity. As an adult, these fears often evolve, taking on a more grave and complex nature - will I recover from this illness? What if I lose my job? Are my loved ones faithful? How will I pay the mounting bills? Death - is it looming closer than I dare to think?

You're not alone. I, Dr. Anthony, have journeyed through these turbulent waters of worry and fear. From the tumultuous waves of childhood anxiety to the undertows of adult apprehensions, I've navigated through this sea of unease. Over time, I've learned to release these anxieties, to break free from these invisible chains, and I am writing this book to share that liberating knowledge with you.

As a school principal, I guard over an ocean of young potential, each wave tainted by the undertow of depression and anxiety. Alongside this role, I am also the pastor of a small local church, nurturing the spiritual growth of a congregation battling the same invisible demons.

Years in education and a lifetime within the warm embrace of the church have given me a panoramic view of the human condition. I've walked the halls of academia and the church's aisles, often discovering that they echo with the same troubled whisper - a cry for understanding, help, and healing. From the innocent faces of my students to the burdened hearts of my congregation, the ripple effects of mental illness pervade every corner of our society.

While I am privileged to hold the titles of principal and pastor, these roles merely serve as platforms for my true calling - being an agent of the Divine Consciousness. I am an advocate of the Almighty, The I AM, Alpha & Omega, Allah - the One by many names - and my mission is clear: to bring solace to the troubled, guidance to the lost, and hope to the despairing.

The question that echoes in my office, in the church, in hushed voices after Sunday service, is always the same: "Why is my life not unfolding as I imagined?" From the sorrow-filled corners of funerals to the strain-ridden faces of families wrestling with their tribulations, I have seen the common thread binding these souls - the constant struggle against forces beyond their control, which consume their lives and shroud their hearts in darkness.

This book is my response to those whispers of despair, a beacon of hope amidst the storm. It is a call to shift our focus from the turbulence around us to the peace within us, a journey into the sanctuary of the 'now.' The pages you are about to turn are not mere words, but the manifestation of my heartfelt prayers, the fruits of my experience, and the distillation of wisdom I've gathered from years of navigating these twin worlds of education and faith.

In the 'Heartbeat of Now,' we free ourselves from the shackles of past regrets and future anxieties. We liberate ourselves from the clutches of depression and invite joy, peace, and presence into our lives. As you embark on this spiritual-practical journey to the power of now, my hope is that you discover the same freedom and serenity that I have found, and I pray this guide illuminates your path towards that freedom.

Welcome, dear reader, to the journey into the Heartbeat of Now.

CHAPTER 1:
UNDERSTANDING ANXIETY
AND DEPRESSION

Anxiety and depression, two terms you've probably heard many times, are more than mere words. They represent real experiences that millions endure, and they're much more than just fleeting feelings of sadness or fear. Let's start our journey by unpacking these terms.

Definition

According to the American Psychiatric Association, anxiety is an emotion characterized by feelings of tension, worried thoughts, and physical changes like increased blood pressure. When these feelings persist and interfere with daily life, they may indicate an anxiety disorder.

Depression, often known as Major Depressive Disorder, is a common and serious medical illness that negatively affects how you feel, the way you think, and how you act. It's characterized by persistent feelings of sadness, loss of interest or pleasure in activities, and can lead to various physical and emotional problems.

Causes and Impact

Anxiety and depression are both complex conditions that can arise from a combination of genetic, biological, environmental, and psychological factors12. Traumatic life experiences, such as the death of a loved one, are well-known triggers, and high-stress environments can also contribute.

In my dual roles as a principal and pastor, I've observed firsthand the impact of these conditions. I've seen bright, energetic students struggle with concentration and lose interest in their favorite activities. I've comforted congregation members who found no joy in life, who grappled with feelings of worthlessness.

The Role of Past Regrets and Future Worries

Anxiety and depression often hinge on time. Regrets about the past and worries about the future can fuel both conditions, leaving individuals stuck in a time other than 'now'. In my years of pastoral counseling, I've noticed a common pattern - individuals often struggle to forgive themselves for past mistakes, and this regret sows the seeds for depression. Similarly, anxiety frequently flares up when individuals excessively worry about the future, about things they cannot control.

From a physical perspective, we often speak of depression and anxiety as conditions rooted in our brain chemistry and our life circumstances, visible in their various debilitating effects. But there's another dimension to these issues, a spiritual aspect that's harder to define, yet deeply influential.

On the spiritual side, I've seen the internal struggles of men, women, and children who grapple with the voices in their heads. The whispers that encourage self-doubt, fear, and hopelessness. Some people describe this as an internal battle, with angels and demons perched on their shoulders. What if I told you that these voices are real, that there is a battle raging for your life?

Now, I understand that scientists and researchers might dismiss this assertion, as it doesn't fit neatly into the empirical frameworks they operate within. Yet, as a pastor, I live in the realm of faith, the realm of the unseen. Ephesians 6:12 in the Bible states, "For our struggle is not against flesh and blood, but against the rulers, against the authorities, against the powers of this dark world and against the spiritual forces of evil in the heavenly realms."

The mission of these dark forces is to keep you mired in depression and anxiety, to prevent you from moving forward and breaking free from the shackles of your past and worries of your future. This book will delve into both the physical and spiritual aspects of anxiety and depression. I do not ask you to take my words at face value, but to engage in your own research, introspection, and journey of understanding.

My prayer for you is that this book resonates with your spirit, and guides you from a place of pain to a position of everlasting peace - peace not as the world gives, but as only Jesus can. As quoted in John 14:27, "Peace I leave with you; my peace I give you. I do not give to you as the world gives. Do not let your hearts be troubled and do not be afraid."

In the chapters to follow, we will chart this dual path to understanding and overcoming anxiety and depression. We will unearth strategies grounded in modern science and spiritual wisdom to bring you into the heart of now, free from the burdens of your past and the fears of your future. I invite you on this journey toward freedom and peace.

CHAPTER 2: WHEN THE BELL RINGS - SCHOOL STORIES OF ANXIETY AND DEPRESSION

As an educational professional, I have been a silent observer to the world of students whose lives are scarred by the crippling forces of anxiety and depression. Behind the lively classrooms and the jovial schoolyard games, there lie hidden narratives of pain, worry, and despair. These stories form the subtext of their lives, subtly influencing their behaviors, attitudes, and academic achievements.

I remember one student, let's call him John, an incredibly bright young man with a passion for mathematics. However, he would often arrive at school looking worn out, disheveled, and aloof. He confided in me one day, revealing a daily struggle with anxiety that would keep him up all night, spiraling in negative thoughts about school, friendships, and life in general. He felt suffocated by the mounting pressure to excel academically, yet socially he felt lost and disconnected. His story is not unique; I've heard echoes of the same fears, the same struggles, from countless others over the years.

The sad truth is that our education system, as it stands, can often contribute to the problem rather than providing the help these children so desperately need. High stakes testing, a relentless focus on academic achievement, and a one-size-fits-all curriculum often exacerbate students' mental health struggles. They feel the burden of expectations, of being constantly measured and evaluated, and the fear of not living up to these standards can be overwhelming.

Research conducted by Suldo et al., (2014) has shown that high-stakes testing has a significant negative impact on students' mental health, contributing to increased stress levels and decreased self-esteem. Another study by Patalay & Gage (2019) shows that the prevalent focus on academic success neglects the critical aspect of mental wellbeing, resulting in an increase in mental health issues among students.

Our approach to education should strive for balance, acknowledging the importance of mental health alongside academic achievement. Schools should be safe spaces for students, where they feel understood, supported, and equipped to deal with their anxieties and fears. We must reshape our educational policies to better address and accommodate the mental health needs of our students.

Maria's Story

There is a story that vividly highlights the heart-wrenching intersection of poverty, mental health, and the education system. This is the story of a fifth-grade girl named Maria. Maria was older than her 11 years. She carried a weight on her shoulders that no child should bear.

Maria was one of five siblings, the oldest in a family overseen by a single mother who worked the night shift at a local factory just to make ends meet. As the oldest, Maria shouldered the responsibility of looking after her younger siblings in the evenings while her mother was at work. This meant cooking meals, ensuring her siblings did their homework, and tucking them into bed, all while trying to juggle her own schoolwork.

During the day, Maria was often found sleeping in class. The strain of her nighttime responsibilities left her exhausted and unable to focus. It wasn't uncommon for her teachers to find her quietly crying when they woke her up. A cloud of sadness seemed to perpetually hang over her, and over time, it became clear that Maria was battling with depression.

Recognizing the severity of Maria's situation, the school counselor, Mrs. Johnson, decided to intervene. She understood that Maria's situation was complex, one that required a solution going beyond the confines of the school walls.

Mrs. Johnson coordinated with local social services to

provide support for Maria's family. She arranged for after-school and evening community programs that Maria's siblings could attend, thus relieving her of some responsibilities. Additionally, Mrs. Johnson established a safe space at school where Maria could talk about her feelings, fears, and frustrations, helping Maria understand her feelings weren't a burden but a shared human experience.

This multi-pronged approach not only addressed Maria's immediate need for rest and relief, but it also began to chip away at the overwhelming weight of depression Maria had been carrying. It was a testament to the profound impact of acknowledging and addressing the often overlooked socio-economic factors that contribute to students' mental health issues.

By sharing Maria's story, I hope to emphasize the vital need for holistic, empathetic approaches in education that take into account each child's unique circumstances. We must recognize and respond to the reality that our students are not just learners in a classroom but human beings navigating complex realities that extend far beyond school walls.

Poverty acts as a magnifying glass, intensifying the prevalence and impact of mental health issues among students. Children from low-income families often face additional stresses at home, further exacerbating their anxiety and depression. Whether it's financial instability, limited access to healthcare, or inadequate nutrition, these hardships form an incessant drone of worry in the back of their minds, making it difficult to focus on school work or build healthy social relationships.

A research study by Reiss (2013) found a direct link between poverty and higher instances of mental health disorders in children and adolescents, reinforcing the fact that socio-economic status is a significant determinant of mental health outcomes.

In communities burdened by poverty, where my school principalships have mostly been, I've observed that parental support, though deeply desired, often lacks consistency. Not because these parents don't want to be there for their children, but because their financial situations don't permit them. Many work hourly jobs, and any time missed means less income, which could jeopardize their ability to pay their bills, meet their needs, and maintain their livelihoods.

Unfortunately, in many of these communities, the internet and digital devices become windows to a world of material opulence that stands in stark contrast to their realities. The exposure to the wealth, lifestyle, and success stories of celebrities can sometimes push individuals further into depression and anxiety. This dangerous fascination with material possessions, and the perceived happiness they bring, can become a heavy chain that weighs down their spirits and blinds them to the beauty of living in the present moment.

Sadly, I've found that both schools and churches often fail to effectively address this issue. There seems to be a prevailing mentality of simply getting by, maintaining the status quo, without taking the time to look beneath the surface and address the unseen struggles that our children and congregants face.

Suicide rates are on the rise, reflecting our collective failure to teach individuals how to let go, to live in the moment, and to channel their creative energies in positive ways. It is a sobering reminder of the urgent need for tools and resources to help people navigate these mental health challenges.

As Jesus said, "The thief comes only to steal and kill and destroy; I have come that they may have life, and have it to the full." While this book isn't about preaching or conversion, it is about providing a roadmap to freedom, equipping you to take control of your mind and daily combat the forces that seek to pull you into darkness.

CHAPTER 3: UNDER THE STEEPLE - CHURCH TALES OF DESPAIR AND HOPE

As a pastor, I stand at the intersection of spiritual faith and the harsh realities of life. While the church steeple points heavenward, the pews are filled with people navigating their earthly struggles, looking for comfort, hope, and understanding.

There are stories of anguish that would shake the faith of the most devout believers: tales of molestation, rape, abuse, murder, financial problems, health issues. Each narrative a poignant reminder of the real hurt that resides within the sanctuary's walls. Among these, "church hurt" stands out as particularly devastating. When the very institution people turn to for refuge becomes the source of their pain, it can lead to a crisis of faith. This is perhaps why Ephesians 6:12 warns us about unseen battles against dark forces.

At times, even prosperity can become a struggle. Riches, while providing material comfort, often fail to insulate against the gnawing emptiness of depression and anxiety. The wealthier members of the congregation, despite their affluence, often grapple with the same existential angst, the same feelings of inadequacy and despair. Their wealth becomes a golden cage, isolating them and making them targets for resentment and envy.

On the other side of the spectrum, there are those who give their last dime in the offering plate, hoping for divine intervention in their dire circumstances. But when their suffering continues unabated, faith falters, and disillusionment sets in. This situation underlines a crisis where the church, instead of being a beacon of hope and a source of comfort, unintentionally exacerbates feelings of despair and hopelessness.

Yet, the church also offers a path towards healing. And this path is paved with faith.

Hebrews 11:1 offers a concise definition of faith: "Now faith is the substance of things hoped for, the evidence of things not seen." Faith empowers us to believe in possibilities beyond our current reality and outside our tangible experiences. It can serve as an effective antidote to depression and anxiety that often stem from a fixation on past regrets and future worries.

The challenge many people face is breaking free from this cycle of hurt, from the relentless replay of painful past memories or the constant dread of an uncertain future. This is where faith coupled with the practice of mindfulness can make a real difference. This combination helps us anchor in the present moment and enables us to understand and respond to our feelings in a healthier way. The power to fight unseen forces doesn't lie in physical weapons but in the spiritual armor we don, primarily the sword of the spirit - the Word of God.

I recall a particular case, one that stands as a powerful illustration of how past regrets and future worries can take a toll on our mental health and spiritual wellness. Let's call this woman Jane.

Jane was a regular churchgoer, but her attendance was inconsistent. She was haunted by a painful past and a persistent worry that history was destined to repeat itself. Jane's mother had passed away after a heated argument between them. Wracked with guilt and convinced that the stress of their altercation had somehow contributed to her mother's death, Jane found herself in the throes of a deep depression. Her nights were filled with nightmares, and her days were hazy, interspersed with periods of fitful sleep. The consequence was a life in shambles, with her work and relationships suffering.

To make matters worse, Jane saw her relationship with her own daughter mirroring the tumultuous one she had with her late mother. The constant fights and misunderstandings brought back painful memories and fed into her anxiety about her daughter's future and their relationship.

Jane's situation was dire, and she sought solace in the church, not dissimilar to how an addict seeks a temporary fix to escape their reality. However, the relief she found was ephemeral, and the cycle of guilt, regret, anxiety, and depression continued.

The key to Jane's healing lay in adopting an attitude of mindfulness and gratitude. I urged Jane to stay grounded in the present, letting go of past regrets and future worries. I encouraged her to forgive herself for her past mistakes and to extend the same grace to her daughter. I reminded her of the importance of releasing the past, not forgetting it, but learning from it and using those lessons to improve the present.

Staying mindful of the present allowed Jane to appreciate her daughter for who she was and to cherish the time they had together, rather than viewing their relationship through the prism of her past regrets. It helped her understand that while she could not control the past or predict the future, she could influence the present by her thoughts, words, and actions. It was not an overnight transformation, but with time, Jane began to experience a sense of peace and a decrease in her depressive symptoms.

This story emphasizes how staying in the power of the now, letting go of the past, and having a grateful heart can lead us to a place of peace and healing. Even in the most challenging circumstances, we can find the strength to move forward by learning from our past and cultivating gratitude for the present moment.

I invite you, dear reader, to accompany me on this journey towards understanding and healing, towards embracing the present moment and moving beyond the limitations of past regrets and future anxieties. My hope is that this exploration of faith, mindfulness, and mental health will not only provide you with valuable insights but also empower you to experience lasting peace and happiness.

CHAPTER 4: THE POWER OF NOW - CONCEPTUAL UNDERSTANDING

What does it mean to live 'in the now'? This concept, deeply embedded in various psychological and spiritual practices, asks us to fully engage with the present moment, unburdened by past regrets and future anxieties. 'Living in the now' does not dismiss the relevance of past experiences or future ambitions. Instead, it encourages us to value and appreciate the present moment for the unique experience it provides.

The origins of this concept can be traced back to various spiritual traditions and psychological theories. From a spiritual perspective, the essence of mindfulness, or 'being in the moment,' is central to practices like Buddhism, Zen, and Taoism. Similarly, Christian worship emphasizes the idea of experiencing God's presence in the here and now, exemplified in the act of Holy Communion. In psychology, mindfulness, a key element in cognitive therapy, urges individuals to focus their attention on the present.

In my work as a school principal and a pastor, I've seen the transformative power of 'living in the now.' In school settings, incorporating mindfulness exercises like deep breathing techniques can dramatically shift a student's focus from ruminating over a past incident or worrying about an upcoming test to concentrating on their breath in the present moment. This simple shift often leads to a reduction in their stress and anxiety levels and increases their capacity to engage with the task at hand.

Similarly, in the church, focusing on worship and the presence of the Holy Spirit helps members to appreciate their current circumstances rather than dwelling on their past mistakes or future worries. In these sacred moments of now, individuals often encounter the unconditional love and grace of God, a love that does not dwell on our shortcomings but embraces us in our imperfections.

My personal experiences have taught me the profound impact of living in the now. Looking back, if I had understood the concept of unconditional love earlier and truly appreciated each moment for what it was, perhaps I would still be married today. Despite our flaws and imperfections, love, acceptance, and gratitude could have sustained our relationship.

Living in the now is not an easy practice, especially when we find ourselves amidst struggles and challenges. However, it's crucial to remember that the battles we fight are often not against people or situations, but against unseen forces. In these moments, our tools are prayer, acceptance, self-forgiveness, gratitude, and the continuous learning and growth that comes from each lived moment. As we navigate these complexities, living in the now can guide us toward a lasting peace.

Remember, 'living in the now' is not about ignoring our past or abandoning the future. Instead, it's about giving our full attention to the present moment, and in doing so, finding a sense of peace and contentment that can be a potent antidote to the stress, anxiety, and unhappiness we often experience. This requires practice and patience, but the rewards - improved mental well-being, deeper relationships, and a heightened appreciation of life's everyday experiences - are well worth the effort.

CHAPTER 5: THE INTERPLAY OF PAST, PRESENT, AND FUTURE

Understanding the interplay between our past, present, and future is essential to cultivating emotional well-being. Each aspect influences our perceptions, attitudes, and behaviors in unique ways, shaping our overall experience of life.

A Lesson from the Past: Understanding Our Emotional Baggage

Our past experiences, particularly those that have been emotionally charged, often linger in our subconscious mind and influence our present behavior and thinking patterns. Whether it's a traumatic incident, a failed relationship, or an unresolved conflict, these experiences can often generate emotional baggage, leading to anxiety, depression, and other mental health issues (Sartorius, 2003).

Learning to identify and understand these past experiences and their impact is the first step in managing their influence on our present and future. Through therapy, mindfulness, and various coping strategies, we can learn to heal from past traumas, releasing their hold on our present lives (D'Andrea & Pole, 2012).

The Future is Now: Redefining Our Relationship with Tomorrow

In many ways, the future is a projection of our present thoughts, feelings, and actions. While it's beneficial to have goals and plans, excessive preoccupation with the future can lead to stress, anxiety, and feelings of being overwhelmed. The key lies in balancing our ambitions for the future with a grounded awareness in the present moment. This mindful approach to planning can result in less anxiety about the future, allowing us to fully engage with our present circumstances (Stoewen, 2017).

The Art of Being: Embracing the Power of Now

As we come to terms with our past and foster a healthier relationship with our future, we free ourselves to embrace the power of now. Living in the present moment, or mindfulness, has been shown to reduce stress, improve mental well-being, and enhance our quality of life (Kabat-Zinn, 1994).

Ms. Clarke

There was a middle-school teacher at one of the schools

I served as principal, let's call her Ms. Clarke. She was an exceptional educator; compassionate, dedicated, and deeply committed to her students. However, she was also haunted by a tumultuous past and plagued by fears of an uncertain future.

Ms. Clarke was the primary caretaker of her ailing father, balancing her demanding job with the responsibility of home healthcare. Additionally, she was grappling with a bitter divorce that had left deep emotional scars. She was exhausted, living in a constant state of worry and fear, and her mental health was visibly deteriorating.

I recall a particularly difficult conversation we had in my office. Tearfully, she confessed her fears of dying alone, her regret over past mistakes, and her anxiety about raising her children in the midst of this emotional turmoil. It was evident that her past traumas and fears for the future were consuming her present, causing her to spiral into depression and anxiety.

Recognizing the depth of her struggle, I suggested that she try a different approach. I explained the concept of 'living in the now', and how this practice could help her to find peace in her daily life. She was skeptical but desperate for change.

We began by incorporating mindful breathing exercises with prayer into her daily routine. She was encouraged to focus on her breath, anchoring herself in the present moment while she prays, thereby gradually detaching from the anxieties of the past and the future. Slowly, she began to see the benefits. She was less reactive, more peaceful, and began to rediscover joy in her everyday tasks.

Together, we worked on embracing gratitude for the present moment. I encouraged her to find joy in her teaching and her children, rather than dwelling on past hurts or future worries.

Over time, with dedication and effort, Ms. Clarke started to transform. Her interaction with her students improved, her relationship with her children deepened, and she even began to enjoy caring for her father, seeing it as an opportunity to express her love rather than a burden.

A couple of years later, Ms. Clarke met a kind man at church revival. They shared a common understanding of living in the present and fell in love. Today, they are happily married. Ms. Clarke, once trapped by her past and terrified of her future, now lives fully in the present, enjoying a peaceful and fulfilling life with her family. Her story serves as a powerful testament to the transformative power of embracing the 'now'.

As we cultivate this mindful presence, we allow ourselves to fully experience and appreciate each moment as it unfolds, unburdened by the past and unhindered by the future. This state of being in the now, accepting and immersing ourselves in the present, is a powerful antidote to the stress and anxiety that often accompany modern life.

CHAPTER 6: SPIRITUAL INSIGHTS INTO LIVING IN THE NOW

From Christianity to Buddhism, Islam to Hinduism, and beyond, the teachings of various religious traditions and spiritual practices offer profound insights into living in the now. While the rituals and customs may differ, the heart of their teachings often points to the same truth - the importance of embracing the present moment.

Christianity

In Christianity, one of the core teachings is about being present and living in the moment, centered on faith in God. In the Bible, Matthew 6:34 states: "Therefore do not worry about tomorrow, for tomorrow will worry about itself. Each day has enough trouble of its own." This verse isn't just about warding off worries, but it's also about being present and appreciating the current moment. Christians are encouraged to surrender their anxieties and fears about the future to God, thus enabling them to be fully engaged in the present.

Julia's Story

Julia was a successful marketing executive who found herself unable to cope with her hectic schedule. Her worrying about the future and regrets about the past were impacting her health and personal life. A friend suggested she join a Bible study group. Through the group, Julia started understanding the teachings of Jesus, especially those on worrying and living in the moment. Julia began to commit 30 minutes every morning to prayer and Bible study, focusing on verses that emphasized trust in God, such as Matthew 6:34: "Therefore do not worry about tomorrow, for tomorrow will worry about itself. Each day has enough trouble of its own." She also started attending weekly church services and participating in a small group Bible study. Through these practices, she learned to 'cast all her anxieties on Him' as suggested in 1 Peter 5:7. This helped her focus less on her worries about the future or past regrets and concentrate on her responsibilities at hand, leading to increased productivity and a more peaceful mind. Gradually, she found herself more calm and present, able to handle her stress better, and lead a more balanced life.

Buddhism

Buddhism's core philosophy is built around mindfulness and awareness of the present moment. The practice of mindfulness, or 'sati' in Pali, is a central part of the

Buddhist path towards nirvana - the state of liberation from suffering. It encourages a direct, experiential understanding of reality as it is in the present moment, without being clouded by judgments or expectations. Through mindfulness, one learns to acknowledge and let go of past regrets and future anxieties, and find peace and contentment in the here and now.

David's Story

David was a university student dealing with anxiety and depression. He had heard about mindfulness meditation and decided to try it. David learned mindfulness meditation from a local Buddhist group. He committed to meditating for 20 minutes each morning, focusing on his breath and allowing his thoughts to pass without judgment. He also attended weekly Dharma talks to deepen his understanding of Buddhist teachings on impermanence and the importance of staying present. Over time, David found himself less anxious about the future and less regretful of the past, leading to improvements in his mental health and academic performance. Over time, he noticed a significant decrease in his anxiety levels and an increase in his ability to concentrate on his studies. He started to live in the moment rather than constantly worrying about the future.

Islam

Islam presents an integral concept known as 'Tawakkul', which can be translated as 'reliance on God.' Muslims are encouraged to put their full trust in Allah's plan, thereby reducing their worries about the past or the future and allowing them to live more fully in the present. Islam also teaches 'Sabr' or patience, which is often practiced during prayer (Salat), where Muslims seek to clear their minds of distractions and focus wholly on their connection with Allah.

Aliyah's Story

Aliyah was a single mother trying to balance work and raising her children. The strain of her responsibilities and the worries about her children's future consumed her. Her local Imam suggested she focus on the Islamic practice of Tawakkul. Aliyah began incorporating the Islamic practice of Tawakkul, or trust in God's plan, into her daily routine. Every day, after her Fajr (dawn) prayer, she would meditate on verses from the Quran that emphasized Tawakkul, such as "And whoever relies upon Allah - then He is sufficient for him." (65:3). This helped her release her anxieties about the future and focus more on her present responsibilities. She also found solace in regular visits to the mosque, where she felt a strong sense of community support. By trusting in Allah's plan, she gradually learned to release her worries about the future and concentrate on her present tasks. This change had a profound effect on her wellbeing and the overall happiness of her family.

Hinduism

The teachings of Hinduism, specifically in the sacred text of the Bhagavad Gita, lay emphasis on 'Karma Yoga' or the path of selfless action. In it, Lord Krishna advises Arjuna to perform his duty without attachment to the results of his actions, saying, "You have the right to work, but never to the fruit of work." This effectively encourages living in the present, focusing on the action at hand without becoming overly concerned with future outcomes.

Ravi's Story

Ravi was a software engineer who felt unsatisfied despite his successful career. After reading the Bhagavad Gita, he started applying the concept of Karma Yoga to his life, focusing on his actions rather than obsessing over outcomes.Ravi started incorporating the teachings of the Bhagavad Gita into his life. He began his day by reading and meditating on verses related to Karma Yoga, the path of selfless action. He particularly focused on the verse "You have a right to perform your prescribed duties, but you are not entitled to the fruits of your actions." (2:47). This practice helped him focus more on his work, find joy in the process, and worry less about the outcomes, thus reducing his stress levels. This shift in perspective allowed him to enjoy his work more, experience less stress, and live more in the present moment.

Taoism

Taoism, an ancient Chinese philosophical and spiritual tradition, advocates for living in harmony with the 'Tao', or the natural way of the universe. Taoism propounds 'wu wei', often translated as 'non-action' or 'effortless action', suggesting a way of life where actions are not forced, but rather, one flows with life as it unfolds in the present moment.

Xiao's Story

Xiao was a small business owner facing stiff competition. He felt constantly on edge, striving to outperform others. He discovered Taoism and started to apply the principle of 'wu wei' - acting in harmony with the flow of life rather than against it. Xiao started his day with Tai Chi, a Taoist practice promoting harmony with the Tao, or the natural flow of life. He also read and reflected on passages from the Tao Te Ching that encourage 'wu wei', or effortless action. This allowed him to make business decisions more in tune with his own values and the needs of his customers, leading to a more satisfying and successful business.

Mindfulness and Meditation Practices

Mindfulness, often associated with Buddhism but increasingly adopted in secular contexts, is a practice of active, open attention on the present. It encourages observing one's thoughts and feelings from a distance, without judging them as good or bad. Similarly, meditation practices, such as transcendental meditation or mindfulness-based stress reduction (MBSR), emphasize focusing attention and eliminating the stream of jumbled thoughts that may be crowding the mind and causing stress.

These spiritual teachings, while diverse in their practices and philosophies, offer similar insights: the value of living in the present moment, and the peace that comes with it.

Sarah's Story

Sarah, a high school teacher, struggled with burnout and a negative self-image. After attending a mindfulness-based stress reduction (MBSR) course, she began to practice mindfulness meditation daily. Sarah began incorporating mindfulness practices into her daily routine. Every morning and evening, she would sit for 15 minutes, focusing on her breath and observing her thoughts without judgment. During the day, she practiced mindful eating and mindful walking, which helped her stay grounded in the present moment. She also attended weekly mindfulness group meetings for support and further learning. Over time, these practices helped her become more aware of her negative thought patterns and let them pass without affecting her self-esteem. She found she was more aware of her negative thought patterns and could let them pass without affecting her self-esteem. This increased her resilience and capacity to handle the stresses of her job and improved her overall mental health.

CHAPTER 7: PRACTICAL STRATEGIES FOR LIVING IN THE NOW

The struggle with anxiety, depression, and stress is often linked to the inability to focus on the present moment. By spending our mental energy reliving the past or forecasting the future, we miss out on the richness of the present. Fortunately, various techniques can assist us in harnessing the power of now. These strategies, grounded in mindfulness practices, cognitive behavioral therapy (CBT), and grounding exercises, can equip us with the skills to live more fully in the present moment.

Mindfulness Techniques

Mindfulness is the process of bringing one's attention to experiences occurring in the present moment, without judgment (Kabat-Zinn, 1994). It is a key element in stress reduction and overall happiness.

1. *Mindful Breathing*: This simple technique involves focusing on your breath, inhaling and exhaling gently,

focusing on each breath as you breathe in and out (Brown & Ryan, 2003).

2. *Mindful Observation*: Choose an object and focus on it for a few minutes. Observe it without judgment, taking note of its color, shape, movement, and other characteristics.

3. *Mindful Listening*: Pay attention to the sounds around you without trying to identify or judge them. This technique helps you anchor in the present moment.

Grounding Exercises

Grounding exercises are techniques that help keep someone in the present. They help reorient a person to the here-and-now and in reality. Grounding skills can be helpful in managing overwhelming feelings or intense anxiety (Rellini et al., 2012).

1. *The 5-4-3-2-1 Technique*: This technique utilizes your five senses to ground you in the present moment. It asks you to acknowledge five things you can see, four things you can touch, three things you can hear, two things you can smell, and one thing you can taste.

2. *Body Scan*: This technique involves paying attention to different parts of your body, from your toes to your head, and noting how they feel in the present moment.

Cognitive Behavioral Techniques

Cognitive behavioral therapy (CBT) is a form of psychological treatment that has been demonstrated to be effective for a range of problems including depression, anxiety disorders, alcohol and drug use problems, marital problems, eating disorders, and severe mental illness (Hofmann, Asnaani, Vonk, Sawyer, & Fang, 2012).

1. *Thought Stopping*: This involves recognizing negative thought patterns and using a distraction technique to interrupt it. This might be a word or phrase, or an action such as snapping a rubber band on your wrist.
2. *Reframing*: This technique helps to change the way you view a situation, and therefore change how you react to it.
3. *Gratitude Journaling*: Keeping a gratitude journal can train our minds to focus on the positive aspects of our day, rather than getting caught up in negative thought patterns.

CHAPTER 8: INTEGRATION OF SPIRITUALITY AND PRACTICALITY

This chapter will delve into the fascinating and enriching process of blending spiritual wisdom with concrete, practical techniques. We will explore how spiritual insights can augment the power of mindfulness practices, grounding exercises, and cognitive behavioral techniques, thereby deepening the experience of living in the now.

Our spiritual beliefs can influence our perception of reality and shape our responses to life events. Meanwhile, practical techniques provide tangible tools to help us navigate our day-to-day existence and manage our mental health. When spirituality and practicality are seamlessly integrated, they can form a comprehensive, holistic approach to living in the present moment.

The interplay between spirituality and practicality is demonstrated in various psychological theories and therapeutic approaches, such as Acceptance and Commitment Therapy (ACT), which integrates mindfulness (a spiritual concept) and behavior change strategies (Hayes et al., 2006). Mindfulness-Based Cognitive Therapy (MBCT) is another example, a program specifically designed to help people who have suffered repeated bouts of depression (Segal et al., 2002).

In my role as a pastor, I guide people who yearn for freedom, towards spiritual practices. The key to confronting unseen forces is prayer. While research and science offer valuable insights and contribute greatly to our understanding, certain aspects of our existence are not completely encapsulated by empirical evidence.

This is where faith comes into play. Faith, while unseen, is the bedrock of belief and trust in something greater. The voices and thoughts that invade your mind are not yours; recognizing this and learning how to combat these intrusive forces is essential to achieving peace and fulfillment.

Relying wholeheartedly on God, trusting Him with all your heart and mind is the key to break every chain that weighs you down, whether physical or spiritual. But the initiative to do better and use the power God has endowed within you lies in your hands.

External factors do not bring true satisfaction or peace. It is the outer world that introduces stress, seeping into our mental well-being and causing depression and anxiety. The real peace comes from God's spirit dwelling within us, a gift bestowed at birth. When we learn to connect with the core of our being and dwell in that spiritual space, we find lasting peace.

But, it's important to remember that staying in that spiritual space requires work. This is what I urge my congregation to strive for every Sunday. The beauty of this journey is that even though I lead, I also follow this path daily. If I don't, I too can fall into the traps set by unseen forces.

It's the merging of spirituality and practicality, the understanding of the battles we wage with unseen forces, and the recognition of our innate power that equips us to live in the present. This is what I strive to impart every Sunday, and this is what I hope will resonate with you.

CHAPTER 9: MINDFUL TEACHING - INTEGRATING THE NOW IN EDUCATION

As an educator and a spiritual guide, my role often extends beyond the confines of administrative tasks and sermon deliveries. One of the most significant aspects of my work revolves around helping students navigate their internal landscapes and supporting them in living in the present.

I've found that the principles of mindfulness can be seamlessly integrated into the educational realm. As such, I've introduced a variety of mindfulness exercises in school, aiming to foster present-focused learning. Here are some of my experiences and tips for educators who wish to do the same:

Creating Safe Spaces: Children, like adults, grapple with a variety of emotions and challenges. Creating safe spaces in school, where children can openly express their feelings, is key. I've noticed that such spaces make students feel valued and heard, encouraging them to focus on the now instead of ruminating over past events or worrying about the future.

Fostering Empathy: Encouraging students to step into others' shoes and consider how they might feel has been an effective tool in teaching them to remain in the present. For instance, post conflict situations, asking students to consider the other party's feelings often calms them and brings them back to the present moment.

Dealing with Deep-rooted Hurt: Deep-rooted hurt, such as instances of child abuse, present unique challenges. However, I've found that focusing on peace and healing, rather than dwelling on past pain, can be instrumental in helping students overcome such experiences. This doesn't mean ignoring the trauma but acknowledging it, addressing it appropriately, and guiding the child towards a path of recovery.

Practicing Mindfulness: Implementing daily mindfulness exercises can help students cultivate a habit of focusing on the present moment. These exercises can range from deep breathing, mindful eating to silent observation of their surroundings.

Cultivating Gratitude: Fostering a culture of gratitude can do wonders in helping students live in the present. Encouraging students to acknowledge and express gratitude for what they have can significantly enhance their focus on the present, and foster positivity.

As an educator, it's crucial to respect the individuality and beliefs of each student. My faith fuels me, but I ensure not to impose my beliefs on my students. Instead, I hope that the love, peace, and compassion I embody will prompt them to inquire and seek their paths.

CHAPTER 10: FAITH IN THE MOMENT - THE POWER OF NOW IN SERMONS AND SERVICES

The principles of living in the now can be traced back to the sacred scriptures. The Bible provides us with a wealth of teachings that encourage us to focus on the present, trust in God's plans, and have faith in His divine timing. As a pastor, integrating these teachings into sermons and church services can offer comfort and guidance to congregants grappling with life's challenges.

Scripture-Based Teachings:

1. **Matthew 6:34**: "Therefore do not worry about tomorrow, for tomorrow will worry about itself. Each day has enough trouble of its own." In this verse, Jesus Himself advises against future-focused worry. This can be a powerful starting point for discussions about the power of living in the now.

2. **Philippians 4:6-7**: "Do not be anxious about anything, but in every situation, by prayer and petition,

with thanksgiving, present your requests to God. And the peace of God, which transcends all understanding, will guard your hearts and your minds in Christ Jesus." This scripture encourages believers to release their anxieties to God, a practice that echoes the present-focused philosophy of mindfulness.

3. **Psalm 46:10**: "Be still, and know that I am God." Encouraging stillness and present moment awareness, this scripture can be used to introduce meditation practices in the church.

4. **Proverbs 3:5-6**: "Trust in the Lord with all your heart and lean not on your own understanding; in all your ways submit to him, and he will make your paths straight." This verse emphasizes faith in God's wisdom over our understanding, promoting trust in God's plans rather than obsessing over our own.

Practical Approaches: Practices From New Jerusalem World Healing Center

1. **Mindful Worship**: One of the most critical pieces in my life as the worship leader, I lead congregants to engage fully in worship services, immersing themselves in the words, music, and communal energy rather than getting caught up in their thoughts.

1. **Prayer & Meditation**: Prayer can be seen as a form of mindfulness, allowing us to connect with God in the present moment. At church we focus on the here and now. The scripture that guides us is John

4: 23 But the hour is coming, and now is, when the true worshipers will worship the Father in spirit and truth; for the Father is seeking such to worship Him. We pray and worship in the now.

2. **Gratitude Practice**: We lead congregants to cultivate an attitude of gratitude. Begin services or Bible studies with a moment of thankfulness for the blessings of the present day. We start services with a great heart prayer and so should you each day you wake up.

3. **Group Discussions**: Facilitate discussions on present-moment awareness during Bible study or fellowship groups. This allows for shared insights and support among the congregation members.

CHAPTER 11: GUIDING THE YOUNG - INSTILLING THE POWER OF NOW IN CHILDREN

Teaching young people the power of now can provide them with crucial coping mechanisms to deal with stress, anxiety, and depression. It's about showing them how to find peace in the moment and developing resilience for the future. As an educator, there are several strategies you can employ to accomplish this.

Teaching Mindfulness in Schools:

1. **Mindful Breathing Exercises**: Start each school day with a mindfulness activity, like a guided breathing exercise. There are numerous videos on YouTube (e.g. Mindful Breathing by Stop, Breathe & Think) that can be played during morning announcements. Such exercises promote calm and focus, setting a positive tone for the day.

2. **Integrating Mindfulness into the Curriculum**: Lessons on mindfulness and living in the present can

be woven into subjects like Health, Social Studies, and even English Language Arts. Teachers can use stories, poems, and classroom discussions to highlight the importance of staying present and aware.

3. **Creating Mindful Spaces**: Designate specific areas in the school where students can practice mindfulness. These can be quiet, comfortable spaces where children can sit, breathe, and be present.

Addressing Anxiety and Depression:

1. **Early Identification**: Teachers and administrators should be trained to identify the early signs of anxiety and depression in students. Early intervention can make a significant difference in a child's mental health journey.

2. **Incorporating Mindfulness into Counseling**: School counselors can use mindfulness-based interventions to help students manage their anxiety or depressive symptoms. Techniques such as grounding exercises and guided imagery can teach students to focus on the present, rather than getting lost in worries about the past or future.

3. **Promoting Open Communication**: Schools should cultivate an environment where mental health is openly discussed. Encourage students to express their feelings and teach them that it's okay to seek help when they're feeling overwhelmed.

Teaching the power of the now to the young generation is an investment in their mental health and their future. By fostering present-moment awareness, we equip them with the tools to break free from cycles of pain and stress, creating a healthier and more resilient generation.

Case Study 1: Mindful Breathing in Baltimore's Patterson High School, USA

In Baltimore's Patterson High School, the Mindful Moment program, developed by the Holistic Life Foundation, was integrated into the school's activities in 2016. The program begins and ends the school day with 15 minutes of yoga and mindfulness meditation, teaching students to focus on their breath and the present moment.

The impact of the program has been substantial. The school reported a significant decrease in suspensions, while the students experienced less stress, improved concentration, and better conflict resolution skills. The practice of mindful breathing has become a normal part of the students' lives, assisting them in remaining present and focused in class and in their personal lives.

References:

1. Suttie, J. (2016). How Mindfulness is Helping Baltimore's Patterson High School. Greater Good Magazine.

Case Study 2: MindUP in the UK

MindUP is a program implemented across a range of UK schools that integrates mindfulness practices into the school day. The program, developed by the Hawn Foundation, consists of 15 lessons, neuroscience, positive psychology, mindful awareness, and social-emotional learning. One of the key practices includes a daily "Brain Break," where students practice deep belly breathing and concentrate on the sounds around them.

Research on the MindUP program found it led to significant improvements in children's behavior and academic performance. Children involved in the program showed better classroom behavior, lower stress, and better math scores compared to peers not involved in the program.

References:

1. Schonert-Reichl, K. A., Oberle, E., Lawlor, M. S., Abbott, D., Thomson, K., Oberlander, T. F., & Diamond, A. (2015). Enhancing cognitive and social–emotional development through a simple-to-administer mindfulness-based school program for elementary school children: a randomized controlled trial. *Developmental psychology*, 51(1), 52.

Case Study 3: 'Calm Classroom' in Chicago Public Schools, USA

The 'Calm Classroom' program has been implemented in more than 3,000 classrooms across Chicago Public Schools. The program involves 3-minute mindfulness techniques that are integrated into the school day at transition times. Techniques include deep breathing, stretching, and relaxation narratives.

An independent evaluation of the program by Lurie Children's Hospital in Chicago found that students who participated in Calm Classroom reported higher levels of patience, calmness, focus, and respect for others. Additionally, teachers reported improved academic performance and behavior in the classroom.

References:

1. Saran, A. (2018). 'Calm Classroom' helps students, teachers refocus. *Chicago Tribune*.
2. H. R. (2019). Lurie Children's Hospital Evaluates Calm Classroom. *Lurie Children's Hospital*.

CHAPTER 12: A PRESENT COMMUNITY - FOSTERING MINDFULNESS IN OUR SOCIAL CIRCLES

Fostering mindfulness in our social circles is a powerful means of constructing robust and supportive communities. The practice of being fully present in the moment and engaging with others around us can transform our relationships and strengthen the ties within our social groups.

The Role of Community in Supporting Mental Health

Community plays an essential role in supporting mental health. Numerous studies have demonstrated that social support can reduce the risk of mental health problems, including depression and anxiety. Moreover, community support has been found to foster resilience and buffer against life's stressors (Holt-Lunstad et al., 2010). In this regard, promoting mindfulness and presence within a community can add another layer of support, teaching individuals how to manage their emotions, decrease stress, and enhance overall well-being.

Incorporating Mindfulness in Community Gatherings

Incorporating mindfulness practices into community gatherings can take various forms. For instance, community prayer or meditation groups can unify people in practicing mindfulness collectively. These gatherings offer a space for individuals to disconnect from their daily worries and focus on their current experiences (Regehr et al., 2013).

Community leaders can also introduce moments of mindful prayer or reflection in community events. These practices can help attendees ground themselves in the present moment, thus enabling them to fully participate in the gathering.

Moreover, mindfulness can be encouraged through discussion groups or workshops, where community members can learn about and discuss spiritual practices that foster mindfulness and share their experiences. Such platforms can provide a supportive environment for individuals to practice mindfulness and deepen their understanding of its benefits (Kang et al., 2013).

The cultivation of mindfulness and presence within a community can have profound effects on its members. As we encourage mindfulness in our social circles, we can create communities that are more compassionate, resilient, and supportive.

CHAPTER 13: YOUR JOURNEY TO THE NOW - A STEP-BY-STEP GUIDE

Embarking on the journey to living in the present moment can be transformative. This journey is not merely about altering one's focus; it's about shifting one's entire perspective on life. This chapter offers a step-by-step guide to begin your journey and help you maintain your path, even amid challenges and setbacks.

Steps to Start Living in the Now

1. **Understanding the Concept**: To begin living in the now, we must first understand what it truly means. Living in the now means focusing on the present moment, rather than dwelling on past regrets or future anxieties (Hofmann et al., 2010).
2. **Self-Assessment**: Reflect on your current state of mind. Consider how often you find yourself stuck in past memories or future worries. Acknowledging

your mental patterns is the first step towards change (Al-Karam & Haque, 2019).

3. **Mindfulness Practices**: Engage in practices that foster mindfulness, such as meditation, breathing exercises, or mindful prayer. These practices can help you become more aware of your current experience and let go of unnecessary thoughts (Ruffault et al., 2017).

4. **Grounding Techniques**: Utilize grounding techniques to bring your focus back to the present moment when you feel your mind wandering. This can involve focusing on your senses or on your breath.

5. **Reframing Techniques**: Cognitive reframing can help you change the way you perceive past regrets and future worries. These techniques often involve identifying negative thoughts and challenging them with more positive or realistic ones (Langer & Moldoveanu, 2000).

Maintaining the Journey: Overcoming Challenges and Setbacks

1. **Practice Regularly**: Consistency is key in maintaining mindfulness. Make it a part of your daily routine, even if it's just for a few minutes each day (Segal et al., 2002).

2. **Embrace the Challenges**: Understand that challenges are a part of the process. It's okay if you find it difficult to focus on the present moment initially.

Be patient with yourself and embrace these challenges as opportunities for growth.

3. **Seek Support**: Don't hesitate to seek support from your community, whether that's through group therapy, prayer groups, or mindfulness workshops. Others can provide valuable insights and encouragement on your journey.

Remember, the journey to living in the now is unique to each individual. Go at your own pace, and remember, the journey itself is a part of living in the now.

Example Schedule for Living in the Now

This is a sample schedule that integrates the steps towards living in the now. It's important to remember that everyone's life and routine are unique, so feel free to adapt this schedule as needed.

Morning:

- 7:00 AM: Wake up, engage in a brief session of gratitude. List three things you are grateful for today.
- 7:15 AM: Mindful breakfast. Be present in the moment, savor each bite without distraction.
- 7:45 AM: 10 minutes of mindful breathing exercise or meditation.

Daytime:

- 12:00 PM: Lunch. Just like breakfast, make this a mindful eating experience.
- 12:30 PM: Five-minute mindful breathing exercise or a mindful prayer.
- 1:00 PM - 5:00 PM: During work or daily chores, practice mindfulness. Notice when your mind wanders off to the past or the future, gently guide it back to the task at hand.

Evening:

- 6:00 PM: Engage in a physical activity you enjoy (like walking, yoga, or playing a sport). Focus on how your body moves and feels during this time.
- 7:00 PM: Dinner. Once again, engage in mindful eating.
- 8:00 PM: Spend quality time with loved ones or engage in a hobby. Practice being fully present during these interactions or activities.
- 9:00 PM: Before bed, engage in a reflective journaling exercise. Write about your successes in staying present today and areas where you found it challenging.

It's important to remember that mindfulness is not just something you do at specific moments during the day, but rather, a way of life. It involves bringing your full attention to whatever you're doing, whether it's eating a meal, working, or spending time with loved ones.

It's also vital to be patient with yourself. If you find it difficult to stay present, gently guide your mind back without judgment. With time and practice, living in the now will become more natural.

Case Study: Embracing the Power of Now in the Classroom

Background:

Anna is a high school teacher in a busy urban school district. She teaches multiple subjects and is constantly juggling lesson planning, grading, parent-teacher conferences, and the unexpected challenges that arise in the classroom. Despite her love for teaching, Anna was feeling overwhelmed by her job, often bringing her work home and losing sleep over it. She was always thinking about the next task or worrying about something she could have done better. She felt like she was missing out on the present moment - not only in her professional life but also in her personal life.

Implementation:

Anna was introduced to the concept of mindfulness and living in the now by a colleague. Intrigued, she started implementing the schedule shared in Chapter 13 of this book. Here's how it looked like for her:

Morning:

- 6:00 AM: Anna woke up and wrote down three things she was grateful for that day - it could be something as simple as the sunshine outside or the fact that she has a job she is passionate about.
- 6:30 AM: During breakfast, she made sure to savor every bite, trying to engage all her senses, instead of grading papers or planning lessons.
- 7:00 AM: Before leaving for school, she spent 10 minutes practicing mindful breathing.

Daytime:

- 11:30 AM: During lunch, Anna made a conscious effort to eat mindfully, even if it was in the staff room surrounded by her colleagues.
- 12:00 PM: Anna found a quiet corner in the school and spent five minutes focusing on her breath.
- Throughout her teaching day: She tried to be fully present with her students, concentrating on the topic she was teaching instead of worrying about the next lesson or the pile of papers she had to grade.

Evening:

- 4:00 PM: After school, Anna went for a run. She focused on the sensation of her feet hitting the pavement, the rhythm of her breath, and the wind against her face.
- 5:30 PM: At dinner, she continued her practice of mindful eating.
- 7:00 PM: During her grading or planning time, she made sure to focus on one task at a time, bringing her mind back whenever it started to wander.
- 9:00 PM: Before bed, Anna journaled about her day, noting the times she was successful in being present and the moments when it was hard.

Outcome:

Over time, Anna noticed significant changes in her life. She felt less stressed and more in control. She also found that she was more patient with her students and colleagues and that she could handle unexpected situations better. Moreover, she was able to leave her work at school and enjoy her personal time. She started to enjoy her job more, feeling more connected to her students and finding joy in their successes. By living in the now, Anna not only improved her mental well-being but also became a better teacher and a happier person.

The transformation in Anna's life didn't go unnoticed.

Seeing her positive changes, many of her colleagues started asking her about her new approach to life. Anna gladly shared her experiences and even started a small mindfulness group at her school, further fostering a sense of community and shared understanding.

Anna's case demonstrates how living in the now can bring about significant positive changes in one's life, both personal and professional. It emphasizes the importance of taking one step at a time and reminds us that mindfulness is a continuous journey, not a destination

CONCLUSION: THE DAWN OF A NEW DAY - ENVISIONING A WORLD LIVING IN THE HEARTBEAT OF NOW

As the final words of this book take shape, I am drawn into a profound reverie, reflecting on the journey that has brought me to this point. The Heartbeat of Now, these three words carry so much more than just the title of this book. They encapsulate a world of wisdom, a lifetime of experiences, and a poignant message for our collective future. But, the journey of writing this book and the wisdom it holds goes beyond my personal experience as a principal, pastor, and human being. It reflects the shared experiences, struggles, victories, and transformative power that comes from truly embracing the present moment, the heartbeat of our existence.

Why "The Heartbeat of Now"? Because our heartbeat, the rhythmic, life-sustaining pulse that keeps us alive, is perhaps the most potent reminder of the present moment. It is constant, always in the now, and to tune into it is to be truly present. Each thump, each rhythm, each pulse, serves as a tangible reminder to focus on ourselves, on our being, on our 'now.' This simple act of awareness, of being grounded in the present, can be the key to unlocking an abundance of peace, serenity, and fulfillment.

I chose to answer a call to share this wisdom because I have seen the impact it can have. I've witnessed it in classrooms and churches, within myself and in those around me. I've seen the transformative power it holds - the power to bring peace, to shatter chains, and to change lives. However, the journey to embracing this wisdom is often peppered with challenges and setbacks. Despite these hurdles, or perhaps because of them, the resulting transformation is profound and deeply rewarding.

Writing this book has been an act of faith. Not faith in the unknown, but faith in the power of the human spirit to overcome adversity, faith in our collective ability to grow and learn, and faith in the transformative power of the present moment. The Heartbeat of Now is more than just a book. It's an invitation - an invitation to start a journey, to dive into the ocean of human potential that lies within each present moment.

I envision a future where this knowledge is wide-spread, where the Heartbeat of Now reverberates in every classroom, every place of worship, every home, and every heart. A future where children are taught the value of the present moment from a young age. A future where work-places and social circles are designed to foster mindfulness and presence. A future where the power of now is not an exception, but a universally recognized, practiced, and treasured norm.

And so, dear reader, my call to action for you is to begin. Start your journey towards living in the Heartbeat of Now. Use the wisdom held in these pages as a guide, but remember, the path is yours, and yours alone to walk. The power is already within you, a hidden treasure waiting to be discovered.

With this book, I hope to plant seeds of change, seeds that grow into strong, towering trees under whose shade future generations can seek refuge. But the responsibility of cultivating these seeds doesn't lie solely with me. It lies with you, dear reader, and with all of us. We are the gardeners of our future, and it is time for us to pick up our tools, roll up our sleeves, and get to work.

I dream of a world where every human being lives in the Heartbeat of Now. A world where each heartbeat resonates with mindfulness, presence, and peace. A world where the rhythmic thump of our hearts serves as a constant reminder to stay rooted in the present moment.

So, let's embark onthis journey together, towards the dawn of a new day, a day lived fully, deeply, and authentically in the Heartbeat of Now.

Here's to the moments yet to come. Here's to the teachers who will guide our children to engage with the world in a present, mindful manner. Here's to the workplaces that will foster mindfulness as an essential tool for productivity and peace. Here's to the community gatherings that will embrace and promote the practices of presence.

Here's to you, dear reader, for you are about to begin an incredible journey. A journey that may have challenges and setbacks but also a journey that promises unparalleled growth and transformation. As you turn the pages of this book, remember, each word is not just meant to be read but lived. Let these pages serve as a beacon, guiding you towards a richer, more fulfilling existence.

Finally, here's to the Heartbeat of Now. To the rhythm that is always with us, guiding us, reminding us of our innate potential. May we all learn to tune into this beat, to dance to its rhythm, to live in its pulse.

As I pen down these last words, my heart is filled with gratitude and hope. Gratitude for the journey that has led me here and hope for the journey that lies ahead of us. This book, The Heartbeat of Now, is not an end, but rather a beginning—a stepping stone towards a future that we can create together.

As you embark on this journey, remember that you are never alone. The beat of your heart, the rhythm of your breath, these are your constant companions, reminding you to stay present, to stay in the now.

In closing, I offer a simple prayer, a beacon of hope. May we all learn to live in the Heartbeat of Now. May we harness the power of the present moment, the power that resides within us. May we cultivate a world where mindfulness, presence, and peace are not merely concepts, but a way of life.

Here's to the dawn of a new day. Here's to a world living in the Heartbeat of Now.

This is my vision. This is our journey. Let's embark on it together, one heartbeat at a time.

In Jesus Name. Amen

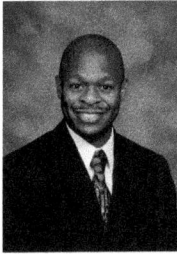

About The
Author

Dr. Anton Anthony, Ed. S, ThD has served in school districts throughout Georgia as a teacher, discipline coordinator, coach, assistant principal, and principal.

He has worked in poverty-stricken schools where most of the population was Title I. He has also worked in schools where parents were highly educated, high-income professionals and business owners. Each school brought its own challenges, but he was able to break through barriers and achieve academic improvement everywhere he went.

Credentials

Dr. Anthony received his Bachelor of Arts with Honors in Business Management from Fort Valley State University in Georgia. He received his Masters of Arts in Teaching at Augusta State University. He later returned to receive a degree in Curriculum and Instruction from Augusta University and received his Educational Specialist add-on in Educational Leadership and Administration, also at Augusta University. He holds his Doctorate in Theology from North Central Theological Seminary. He is a licensed educator and real estate broker with the State of Georgia.

Career

He began his educational career as a reading specialist in Burke County, Georgia schools. He was moved into the 7th grade English/Language Arts program (ELA), where he experienced his first real taste of educational success. His class achieved the highest passing percentage, and he was given an award to recognize his achievement.

After spending a second year at the middle school where he began his career, he asked for a position as a coach at an alternative school in that same district. Former teacher of the year for the school, he was allowed to become the coach, discipline coordinator, and reading instructor.

From those positions, he would become an assistant principal and principal. He is currently a public school principal in Georgia to be closer to his children.

Current Status

Mr. Anthony currently lives in Georgia. He is one of the most active administrators on social media and looks forward to bringing his vision of AA STEAM & Entrepreneurship Academy to life.

REFERENCES

1. Al-Karam, C. Y., & Haque, A. (2019). Mental health concepts in Southeast Asia: diagnostic considerations and treatment implications. Psychology, Health & Medicine, 24(1), 63-76.

2. American Psychiatric Association. (2013). Diagnostic and statistical manual of mental disorders (5th ed.). https://www.psychiatry.org/psychiatrists/practice/dsm

3. Bell, D. (2013). Practical Spirituality: The spiritual basis of nonviolent communication. PuddleDancer Press.

4. Black, D. S., & Fernando, R. (2014). Mindfulness training and classroom behavior among lower-income and ethnic minority elementary school children. Journal of Child and Family Studies, 23(7), 1242-1246.

5. Brown, K. W., & Ryan, R. M. (2003). The benefits of being present: mindfulness and its role in psychological well-being. Journal of personality and social psychology, 84(4), 822–848. doi:10.1037/0022-3514.84.4.822

6. D'Andrea, W., & Pole, N. (2012). A naturalistic study of the relation of psychotherapy process to changes in symptoms, information processing, and physiological activity in complex trauma. Psychological trauma: theory, research, practice, and policy, 4(4), 438.

7. Greenberg, M. T., & Harris, A. R. (2012). Nurturing mindfulness in children and youth: Current state of research. Child development perspectives, 6(2), 161-166.

8. Gunaratana, Henepola. "Mindfulness in Plain English." Wisdom Publications, 2002.

9. Hayes, S. C., Luoma, J. B., Bond, F. W., Masuda, A., & Lillis, J. (2006). Acceptance and Commitment Therapy: Model, processes and outcomes. Behavior Research and Therapy, 44(1), 1-25.

10. Hayes, S. C., & Plumb, J. C. (2007). Mindfulness from the bottom up: Providing an inductive framework for understanding mindfulness processes and their application to human suffering. Psychological Inquiry, 18(4), 242-248.

11. Hicks, E. K., Hicks, J., & Hicks, S. (1999). A new beginning II: A personal handbook to enhance your life, liberty and pursuit of happiness. Hay House, Inc.

12. Hofmann, S. G., Asnaani, A., Vonk, I. J., Sawyer, A. T., & Fang, A. (2012). The Efficacy of Cognitive Behavioral Therapy: A Review of Meta-analyses. Cognitive therapy and research, 36(5), 427–440. doi:10.1007/s10608-012-9476-1

13. Hofmann, S. G., Sawyer, A. T., Witt, A. A., & Oh, D. (2010). The effect of mindfulness-based therapy on anxiety and depression: A meta-analytic review. Journal of Consulting and Clinical Psychology, 78(2), 169–183.

14. Holt-Lunstad, J., Smith, T. B., & Layton, J. B. (2010). Social Relationships and Mortality Risk: A Meta-analytic Review. PLoS Medicine, 7(7), e1000316.

15. Kabat-Zinn, J. (1994). Wherever you go, there you are: Mindfulness meditation in everyday life. Hyperion.

16. Kabat-Zinn, J. (2009). Full catastrophe living: Using the wisdom of your body and mind to face stress, pain, and illness. Delta.

17. Kabat-Zinn, J. (2009). Wherever you go, there you are: Mindfulness meditation in everyday life. Hachette Books.

18. Koenig, H.G., King, D., & Carson, V.B. (2012). Handbook of Religion and Health. Oxford University Press.

19. "Matthew 6:34." BibleGateway. Accessed on [Date].

20. "Quran, 7:189." Quran.com. Accessed on [Date].

21. Mitchell, Stephen. "Bhagavad Gita: A New Translation." Harmony, 2002.

22. National Institute of Mental Health. (2018). Depres-

sion. https://www.nimh.nih.gov/health/topics/depression/index.shtml

23. Neff, K. D., & Dahm, K. A. (2015). Self-compassion: What it is, what it does, and how it relates to mindfulness. In B. D. Ostafin, M. D. Robinson, & B. P. Meier (Eds.), Handbook of mindfulness and self-regulation (p. 121–137). Springer.

24. Patalay, P., & Gage, S. H. (2019). Changes in millennial adolescent mental health and health-related behaviours over 10 years: a population cohort comparison study. International Journal of Epidemiology, 48(5), 1650–1664. https://doi.org/10.1093/ije/dyz006

25. Reiss, F. (2013). Socioeconomic inequalities and mental health problems in children and adolescents: A systematic review. Social Science & Medicine, 90, 24-31.

26. Sartorius, N. (2003). The impact of mental illness on the individual and society. Psychiatria Danubina, 15(1-2), 4-8.

27. Segal, Z. V., Williams, J. M. G., & Teasdale, J. D. (2018). Mindfulness-based cognitive therapy for depression. Guilford Publications.

28. Smith, T. B., Bartz, J., & Richards, P. S. (2007). Outcomes of religious and spiritual adaptations to psychotherapy: A meta-analytic review. Psychotherapy Research, 17(6), 643-655.

29. Stanley, M.A., Bush, A.L., Camp, M.E., Jameson, J.P., Phillips, L.L., Barber, C.R., Zeno, D., Lomax, J.W., & Cully, J.A. (2011). Older adults' preferences for religion/spirituality in treatment for anxiety and depression. Aging Ment Health, 15(3), 334-343.

30. Stoewen, D. L. (2017). Dimensions of wellness: Change your habits, change your life. The Canadian Veterinary Journal, 58(8), 861.

31. Suldo, S. M., Thalji, A., & Ferron, J. (2011). Longitudinal academic outcomes predicted by early adolescents' subjective well-being, psychopathology, and mental health status yielded from a dual factor model. The Journal of Positive Psychology, 6(1), 17–30. https://doi.org/10.1080/17439760.2010.536774

32. "Tao Te Ching." Translated by Stephen Addiss and Stanley Lombardo. Hackett Publishing Company, 1993.

33. Thich Nhat Hanh. (1999). The Miracle of Mindfulness: An Introduction to the Practice of Meditation. Beacon Press.

34. Thieleman, K., Cacciatore, J., & Hill, P. W. (2014). Traumatic bereavement and mindfulness: A preliminary study of mental health outcomes using the ATTEND Model. Clinical Social Work Journal, 42(3), 260-268.

35. Tolle, E. (2004). The power of now: A guide to spiritual enlightenment. New World Library.

36. W. R. Miller & B. L. Fredrickson, "Affective Generativity and Spiritual Tranformation," Journal of Psychology and Christianity 23 (2004): 291–301.

www.ingramcontent.com/pod-product-compliance
Lightning Source LLC
Chambersburg PA
CBHW071246020426
42333CB00015B/1653